Best exercise For Bedridden Patients

Engage in simple limb exercises to promote circulation and flexibility.

By
Ellie Grace

Table of Content

Best Exercise for Bedridden people

Introduction

Living with out of commission conditions represents various difficulties for people. The effect goes past actual limits, affecting profound prosperity, social associations, and generally speaking personal satisfaction. Tending to the diverse parts of this present circumstance requires an exhaustive methodology that includes clinical consideration, mental help, and way of life changes.

Right off the bat, the clinical viewpoint assumes a significant part in guaranteeing the prosperity of disabled people. Customary wellbeing evaluations, observing imperative signs, and forestalling inconveniences, for example, pressure ulcers are fundamental. Talented nursing care, given by medical services experts, becomes foremost to keep up with cleanliness, manage prescriptions, and address any developing clinical necessities. Cooperative endeavors between medical services suppliers, patients, and their families are vital in formulating powerful consideration plans custom fitted to the particular requirements of every person.

Profound prosperity is frequently ignored however is similarly huge. The mental cost of being out of commission can be significant, prompting sensations of separation, despondency, and uneasiness. Laying out an emotionally supportive network that incorporates psychological wellness experts, relatives, and companions is fundamental. Taking part in exercises that advance mental excitement, like perusing, paying attention to music, or even virtual social associations, can contribute emphatically to one's personal state.

Besides, keeping a feeling of direction is urgent for laid up people. Chasing after side interests that can be adjusted to the bound space, like composition, composing, or mastering new abilities on the web, can give a feeling of achievement and motivation. Furthermore, innovation assumes an essential part in interfacing disabled people with the rest of the world. Video calls, virtual entertainment, and online networks offer roads for keeping up with social associations, diminishing sensations of depression.

The actual limits of being disabled require way of life changes. Particular hardware, for example, movable beds, pressure-alleviating beddings, and portability helps, can upgrade solace and forestall entanglements. Besides, legitimate sustenance is pivotal for keeping up with generally wellbeing and forestalling muscle decay. Teaming up with nutritionists to make adjusted dinner plans custom fitted to individual necessities is fundamental.

Integrating active recuperation into the everyday schedule is another crucial viewpoint. Laid up people face the gamble of muscle shortcoming and joint solidness. Basic activities, directed by physiotherapists, can assist with keeping up with versatility, further develop course, and forestall optional medical problems. Versatile yoga or extending schedules, altered for bed use, can likewise add to actual prosperity.

Monetary contemplations add one more layer of intricacy to the existences of incapacitated people. The expense of clinical consideration, specific hardware, and potential home adjustments can be huge. Exploring protection, investigating monetary help projects, and looking for local area support become fundamental parts of dealing with the monetary part of an incapacitated way of life.

Family guardians assume an instrumental part in the existences of out of commission people. The obligations they shoulder, including actual consideration, basic reassurance, and backing for clinical necessities, can overpower. Giving assets and backing to parental figures is pivotal to forestall burnout and guarantee the prosperity of both the guardian and the disabled person.

Establishing a comprehensive and available climate is crucial for society to help disabled people. Public spaces, transportation, and sporting offices ought to be planned in light of availability. Bringing issues to light about the difficulties l

Chapter1
Neck stretches

Extending your neck is significant for keeping up with adaptability and decreasing strain. Here are some neck extends you can integrate into your daily practice:

Neck Slant:

Gradually slant your head aside, bringing your ear toward your shoulder.
Hold for 15-30 seconds.
Rehash on the opposite side.

Neck Revolution:

Tenderly turn your head aside, investigating your shoulder.
Hold for 15-30 seconds.
Rehash on the opposite side.

Neck Flexion:

Gradually lower your jawline towards your chest, feeling a stretch toward the rear of your neck.
Hold for 15-30 seconds.

Neck Expansion:

Slant your head in reverse, turning upward towards the roof.
Hold for 15-30 seconds.
Side-to-Side Head Slant your head aside, bringing your ear towards your shoulder. Then, at that point, tenderly slant your head to the opposite side.
Rehash for 1-2 minutes.

Shoulder Rolls:

Roll your shoulders in reverse in a round movement.
This helps discharge strain in the neck and upper back.
Jawline Tucks:

Sit or remain with a straight spine.
Gradually fold your jaw toward your chest, making a
twofold jaw.
Hold for a couple of moments, then, at that point,
discharge.

Situated Neck Stretch:

Sit serenely with your back straight.
Put your right hand on the left half of your head and
delicately pull, feeling a stretch on the right half of your
neck.
Hold for 15-30 seconds.
Rehash on the opposite side.

Neck and Shoulder Stretch:

Catch your hands behind your back and fix your arms.
Lift your arms somewhat, opening your chest and
extending your neck.
Ear-to-Shoulder Stretch:

Delicately bring your ear towards your shoulder, feeling
a stretch on the contrary side.
Hold for 15-30 seconds.
Rehash on the opposite side.
Make sure to play out these stretches gradually and
easily, keeping away from any unexpected
developments. On the off chance that you experience
torment or uneasiness, pause and talk with a medical

services proficient. Integrating these stretches into your routine can assist with further developing neck adaptability and diminish firmness

Chapter2
Shoulder rolls

an apparently basic and frequently disregarded work out, harbor a universe of advantages for the human body. This elegant development includes the turn of shoulders in roundabout movements, making a liquid and controlled grouping. Notwithstanding its clear effortlessness, shoulder rolls contribute altogether to generally wellbeing, prosperity, and actual execution. In this extensive investigation, we will dig into the life systems of the shoulder, the mechanics of shoulder rolls, their authentic importance, and the bunch benefits they offer.

I. Life systems of the Shoulder:

Understanding the life systems of the shoulder is critical for valuing the effect of shoulder rolls on the body. The shoulder is an intricate joint including the homers (upper arm bone), scapula (shoulder bone), and clavicle (collarbone). The glen humeral joint, where the homers interfaces with the scapula, takes into consideration an extensive variety of movement. Tendons, ligaments, and muscles, like the deltoids and rotator sleeve, assume imperative parts in balancing out and working with development inside the shoulder joint.

II. Mechanics of Shoulder Rolls:

Shoulder rolls include a repeating movement that draws in different muscles and joints inside the shoulder complex. The development normally begins with a delicate lift of the shoulders towards the ears, trailed by a smooth in reverse pivot, lastly, a descending and forward movement. This round arrangement advances adaptability, portability, and further developed blood dissemination inside the shoulder joints and encompassing muscles.

III. Verifiable Importance:

The underlying foundations of shoulder rolls follow back to old practices and teaches that focus on body mindfulness and prosperity. Customary development based exercises, for example, yoga and Kendo, consolidate shoulder rolls as indispensable parts of their schedules. These activities were perceived for their capacity to improve energy stream, discharge pressure, and advance mental lucidity. Shoulder rolls were not simply actual activities however were embraced for their comprehensive advantages, encouraging an association between the body, psyche, and soul.

IV. Advantages of Shoulder Rolls:

a. Further developed Adaptability and Scope of Movement:
Shoulder rolls focus on the muscles and tendons around the shoulder joint, advancing expanded adaptability and a more extensive scope of movement. Normal practice can mitigate solidness and improve the general versatility of the shoulders, forestalling the advancement of ongoing circumstances like frozen shoulder.

b. Upgraded Flow and Joint Oil:

The round movement of shoulder rolls animates blood stream to the shoulder region, conveying oxygen and supplements to the muscles and joints. Furthermore, this development disseminates synovial liquid inside the joint, working with smoother and more easy developments.

c. Stress Decrease and Unwinding:

The musical and dull nature of shoulder rolls initiates a feeling of quiet and unwinding. This exercise has been integrated into pressure the executives programs, as it urges people to zero in on the current second and delivery strain put away in the shoulders and neck.

d. Act Improvement:

Shoulder rolls add to more readily pose by focusing on the muscles that help the spine and upper back. Fortifying these muscles balances the adverse consequences of delayed sitting and slumping, advancing an upstanding and adjusted act.

e. Injury Counteraction and Recovery:

Standard consideration of shoulder rolls in a wellness routine can act as a proactive measure against shoulder wounds. Moreover, for people recuperating from shoulder-related wounds or medical procedures, controlled shoulder roll activities can support restoration by advancing delicate development and forestalling firmness.

f. Mind-Body Association:

The conscious and careful execution of shoulder rolls cultivates a more profound association between the body and brain. This psyche body mindfulness is fundamental to rehearses like yoga and care reflection, where the attention on breath and development upgrades in general prosperity.

V. Integrating Shoulder Rolls into Your Everyday practice:

Whether you are a competitor, a wellness lover, or somebody hoping to work on in general wellbeing, coordinating shoulder rolls into your routine is a straightforward yet powerful methodology. These activities can be proceeded as independent stretches or integrated into warm-up and cool down schedules. It's crucial for start with delicate developments and steadily increment the power to keep away from strain.

VI. Varieties of Shoulder Rolls:

To take care of assorted wellness levels and inclinations, there are a few varieties of shoulder rolls. These may incorporate situated or standing varieties, slow and controlled developments for care, or dynamic and fiery rolls for heating up before additional extraordinary proactive tasks. Investigating these varieties permits people to fit their shoulder roll practice to their particular necessities and objectives.

VII. Conclusion:

All in all, shoulder rolls are something beyond a progression of roundabout developments; they address an all encompassing way to deal with wellbeing and prosperity. With establishes in old practices and a large number of advantages for the cutting edge individual, shoulder rolls merit a spot in everybody's wellness collection. Whether you are looking for further developed adaptability, stress decrease, or injury counteraction, integrating shoulder rolls into your routine can add to a better and more adjusted way of life. Embrace the polish and straightforwardness of shoulder rolls to open the maximum capacity of this ageless exercise.

Chapter 3
Ankle circle

Lower leg circles are a straightforward yet successful activity that includes pivoting the lower leg joint in a round movement. This apparently fundamental development holds various advantages for people of any age and movement levels. In this complete investigation, we will dive into the life structures of the lower leg, the significance of lower leg versatility, the particular benefits of lower leg circles, and different procedures and applications for integrating this activity into everyday schedules.

Life structures of the Lower leg:

Prior to digging into lower leg circles, it's vital to comprehend the life structures of the lower leg joint. The lower leg is a mind boggling joint involving three fundamental bones: the tibia, fibula, and bone. Tendons, ligaments, and muscles work as one to give solidness and work with development. The lower leg joint essentially permits dorsiflexion (lifting the foot toward the shin) and plantar flexion (pointing the foot away from the shin), as well as reversal and eversion (rotational developments).

Significance of Lower leg Versatility:

Lower leg versatility assumes a vital part in generally speaking development and usefulness. Restricted lower leg versatility can prompt compensatory developments, influencing nearby joints like the knee, hip, and lower back. Deficient lower leg adaptability might add to ill-advised walk examples, unsteadiness, and an expanded gamble of wounds. Participating in practices that improve lower leg portability, for example, lower leg circles, can moderate these issues and advance in general joint wellbeing.

Advantages of Lower leg Circles:

Further developed Scope of Movement (ROM): Lower leg circles effectively draw in the lower leg joint through its full scope of movement. Ordinary practice can improve adaptability, considering smoother and more effective development during exercises like strolling, running, and hopping.

Joint Grease:

The round movement of lower leg circles advances synovial liquid course inside the joint. This grease diminishes grinding, limiting mileage on the articular surfaces and supporting joint wellbeing.

Counteraction of Firmness:

Stationary ways of life or drawn out times of fixed status can add to joint firmness. Lower leg circles act as a magnificent unique stretch, supporting the avoidance of firmness and keeping up with joint gracefulness.

Upgraded Proprioception:

Lower leg circles animate the proprioceptive receptors around the joint, working on the body's consciousness of its situation in space. This increased proprioception adds to all the more likely equilibrium and coordination, decreasing the gamble of falls and wounds.

Restoration and Injury Anticipation:
For people recuperating from lower leg wounds or medical procedures, lower leg circles can be a significant recovery instrument. The controlled development reestablishes capability, fortify supporting muscles, and forestall future wounds.

Strategies for Performing Lower leg Circles:

Performing lower leg circles is a clear activity that can be adjusted to different wellness levels. Here is a bit by bit guide:

Situated Lower leg Circles:

Sit serenely on a seat or the floor with legs expanded.
Lift one foot off the ground.
Turn the lower leg in a roundabout movement, first clockwise and afterward counterclockwise.
Rehash the movement for 10-15 reiterations and change to the next lower leg.

Standing Lower leg Circles:

Stand with feet hip-width separated.
Lift one foot somewhat off the ground.
Pivot the lower leg clockwise and afterward counterclockwise.
Perform 10-15 circles toward every path prior to changing to the next lower leg.
Dynamic Lower leg Circles:

Integrate lower leg circles into dynamic warm-up schedules before proactive tasks.

Consolidate lower leg circles with other joint developments to set up the whole lower body for work out.

Opposition Band Lower leg Circles:

Secure an obstruction band around a proper point and circle it around the highest point of the foot.
Perform lower leg circles against the obstruction of the band to add a component of solidarity preparing to the activity.
Utilizations of Lower leg Circles:

Warm-Up Everyday practice:

Incorporate lower leg circles in your warm-up everyday practice to set up the lower legs for more serious actual work. This can be particularly advantageous prior to participating in sports or weight-bearing activities.

Recuperation and Restoration:

Lower leg circles are significant in post-injury or post-medical procedure restoration programs. They assist with recapturing portability, fortify the encompassing muscles, and work with a smooth recuperation process.

Work area Activities:

People with stationary positions can perform lower leg circles circumspectly under their work areas. This gives a method for fighting firmness and advancing dissemination during extensive stretches of sitting.

Equilibrium and Security Preparing:

Integrate lower leg circles into balance activities to improve solidness. Performing circles on one foot difficulties the proprioceptive framework, adding to further developed balance over the long haul.

Athletic Execution Improvement:

Competitors in different games, like artists, sprinters, and b-ball players, can profit from incorporating lower leg circles in their preparation schedules. Further developed lower leg versatility can mean upgraded execution and diminished injury risk.

Conclusion:

All in all, lower leg circles offer a bunch of advantages that stretch out past the straightforwardness of their development. By grasping the life systems of the lower leg, perceiving the significance of lower leg portability, and integrating lower leg circles into ordinary schedules, people can advance joint wellbeing, forestall wounds, and upgrade generally actual prosperity. Whether as a warm-up, a recuperation instrument, or a piece of restoration programs, lower leg circles stand as a flexible and open activity with the possibility to decidedly influence people across different ways of life and wellness levels

Chapter4
Seated leg lifts

are a flexible and compelling activity that objectives different muscle bunches in the lower body. Whether you are a wellness lover hoping to fortify your legs, a competitor planning to upgrade execution, or somebody looking for restoration after a physical issue, situated leg lifts offer a significant expansion to your gym routine daily practice. This complete aide investigates the advantages, appropriate methods, and varieties of situated leg lifts, revealing insight into how this exercise can add to generally wellness and prosperity.

Advantages of Situated Leg Lifts:

Muscle Initiation:
Situated leg lifts essentially draw in muscles in the quadriceps, hamstrings, and hip flexors. This designated enactment further develops muscle strength, tone, and perseverance in the lower limits.

Center Security:
While situated leg lifts fundamentally center around the lower body, they likewise require a level of center security to keep an upstanding stance. This commitment of the center muscles adds to generally speaking solidness and equilibrium.

Joint Portability:
The controlled development of situated leg lifts advances joint portability in the hip and knee joints.

This can be especially useful for people managing firmness or trying to upgrade adaptability.

Low-Effect Exercise:

Situated leg lifts are a low-influence work out, making them reasonable for people with joint worries or those recuperating from wounds. The controlled idea of the development limits weight on the joints while as yet giving a successful exercise.

Adaptability in Preparing:

Situated leg lifts can be adjusted to different wellness levels, from fledglings to cutting edge competitors. By changing the force, reiterations, or integrating extra obstruction, people can fit the activity to their particular necessities and objectives.

Methods for Situated Leg Lifts:

Setup:

Sit on a tough seat or seat with your back straight and feet level on the floor.
Put your hands on the sides of the seat or clutch the edges for help.

Leg Lift Execution:

Lift one leg straight out before you, drawing in the quadriceps.
Hold the lifted leg briefly, guaranteeing control and steadiness.
Gradually further the leg back down to the beginning position.
Rehash the development on the contrary leg.
Breathing:

Breathe in as you lift your leg.
Breathe out as you bring down your leg.

Posture:

Keep an upstanding stance all through the activity.
Try not to recline or slumping to guarantee appropriate
muscle commitment.
Varieties of Situated Leg Lifts:

Obstruction Groups:

Present obstruction groups around your lower legs or
thighs to add additional test and focus on the muscles
from various points.

Lower leg Loads:

Tie on lower leg loads to expand the opposition and
increase the exercise, advancing strength and muscle
perseverance.

Isometric Holds:

Lift one leg and stand firm on it in the raised footing for
a lengthy period to consolidate isometric constrictions,
improving muscle perseverance.

Rotating Leg Lifts:

Lift one leg and afterward the other in a liquid, rotating
movement to keep a ceaseless commitment of the lower
body muscles.
Situated Leg Lifts with Turn:

Consolidate situated leg lifts with a rotational development, drawing in the center muscles to a greater extent.

Tips for a Powerful Situated Leg Lift Exercise:

Begin Slowly:

On the off chance that you are new to situated leg lifts, start with a couple of reiterations and step by step increment as your solidarity and perseverance get to the next level.

Center around Structure:

Focus on legitimate structure over the quantity of reiterations. This guarantees that you are focusing on the right muscles and limiting the gamble of injury.

Pay attention to Your Body:

Focus on any uneasiness or agony during the activity. On the off chance that you experience torment, stop the development and counsel a wellness expert or medical care supplier.

Remember for a Fair Daily practice:

While situated leg lifts offer various advantages, integrating them into a balanced work-out schedule that incorporates cardiovascular, strength, and adaptability preparing is fundamental for in general wellness.

Conclusion:

Situated leg lifts are an important expansion to any wellness routine, giving a scope of advantages from muscle enactment to joint versatility. Whether you are recuperating from a physical issue, expecting to fortify your lower body, or hoping to improve athletic execution, situated leg lifts offer a flexible and open arrangement. By grasping the legitimate methods, varieties, and integrating them into a decent exercise routine daily schedule, you can bridle the maximum capacity of situated leg lifts for further developed strength, solidness, and in general well-being. Leg lifts.

Chapter5
Deep breathing exercise

In the high speed, stress-ridden world we occupy today, the quest for all encompassing prosperity has become progressively vital. Among the plenty of wellbeing rehearses accessible, profound breathing activities have arisen as an integral asset for advancing mental, close to home, and actual wellbeing. This extensive investigation digs into the beginnings, advantages, methods, and logical underpinnings of profound breathing activities, revealing insight into their groundbreaking potential.

I. Authentic Roots:

Profound breathing activities have antiquated roots, following back to different pondering customs and recuperating rehearses. In Eastern societies, disciplines like yoga and Jujitsu underscore the significance of breath control for of accomplishing amicability among psyche and body. Pranayama, a yogic work on starting from old India, explicitly centers around dominating the breath to accomplish mental lucidity and profound illumination. In the West, profound breathing has been basic to care and contemplation rehearses, with its restorative advantages perceived in different social and otherworldly settings.

II. Physiological Establishments:

Understanding the physiological components behind profound breathing gives knowledge into its groundbreaking impacts on the body. The autonomic sensory system, including the thoughtful and parasympathetic branches, assumes a crucial part. Profound breathing actuates the parasympathetic sensory system, setting off the unwinding reaction and balancing the pressure initiating impacts of the thoughtful framework. This physiological shift prompts diminished pulse, brought down circulatory strain, and upgraded by and large prosperity.

III. Mental Effect:

The association among breath and feelings is significant, making profound breathing activities an intense device for overseeing mental prosperity. The diaphragmatic breathing quality of profound breathing connects with the vague nerve, affecting the arrival of synapses like serotonin and gamma-amino butyric corrosive (GABA). These neurochemical changes add to decreased uneasiness, further developed temperament, and upgraded mental capability. Integrating profound breathing into everyday schedules encourages close to home flexibility and develops a careful consciousness of one's psychological state.

IV. Stress Decrease:

In a world portrayed by ongoing pressure, the effortlessness and openness of profound breathing make it a significant remedy. The pressure reaction, set apart by the arrival of cortisol and adrenaline, can be regulated through controlled breathing procedures. Research reliably shows the viability of profound taking in diminishing feelings of anxiety, offering people a useful and normal method for dealing with the requests of current life. Utilizing profound breathing as a proactive pressure the board device engages people to explore difficulties with levelheadedness and strength.

V. Mental Advantages:

Past its effect on pressure and feelings, profound breathing activities apply significant mental advantages. Oxygen is fundamental for mind capability, and controlled breathing upgrades oxygenation. This upgraded oxygen supply works on mental execution, focus, and memory. Profound breathing likewise empowers a shift from the default mode organization, related with mind-meandering and self-referential contemplations, to the undertaking positive organization, advancing centered consideration and mental clearness.

VI. Improving Rest Quality:

Quality rest is vital to by and large prosperity, and profound breathing arises as a characteristic and powerful guide for further developing rest. The unwinding reaction initiated by profound breathing decidedly impacts the rest wake cycle, advancing a condition of quiet helpful for relaxing rest. Integrating profound breathing activities into sleep time schedules can ease a sleeping disorder, decrease rest unsettling influences, and upgrade the general nature of rest, adding to supported physical and mental imperativeness.

VII. Useful Procedures:

A few profound breathing procedures take care of various inclinations and settings. Diaphragmatic breathing, box breathing, and the 4-7-8 procedure are among the generally polished techniques. Diaphragmatic breathing includes breathing in profoundly through the nose, permitting the stomach to extend completely, and breathing out leisurely through tightened lips. Box breathing, promoted by the military, stresses breathing in, holding, breathing out, and stopping for equivalent lengths. The 4-7-8 strategy includes breathing in for a count of four, holding the breath for seven counts, and breathing out discernibly for eight counts. Exploring different avenues regarding these procedures permits people to find the one that resounds best with their inclinations and requirements.

VIII. Developing Care:

Profound breathing fills in as a passage to care — a consciousness of the current second without judgment. By mooring regard for the breath, people can develop an uplifted feeling of mindfulness, cultivating a profound association with the present. This care practice reaches out past conventional contemplation meetings, pervading everyday exercises and connections. The coordination of care through profound breathing causes a significant change in one's point of view, advancing a more adjusted and satisfying presence.

IX. Application in Different Settings:

The flexibility of profound breathing renders it relevant in assorted settings and settings. From corporate meeting rooms to homerooms, medical clinics to athletic fields, people from varying backgrounds can bridle the advantages of profound relaxing. Work environment health programs progressively consolidate profound breathing activities to upgrade representative efficiency and prosperity. In instructive settings, understudies and teachers the same advantage from consolidating brief breathing activities to reduce pressure and further develop center. The flexibility of profound breathing makes it a widespread and open device for encouraging a culture of prosperity in different conditions.

X. Customized Approaches:

While profound breathing activities offer a generally open way to prosperity, personalization is vital to boosting their viability. People might reverberate with explicit strategies, terms, or frequencies. Fitting profound breathing practices to line up with individual inclinations and timetables guarantees more prominent adherence and maintainability. Coordinating profound breathing into existing schedules, whether during drives, breaks, or before sleep time, improves the probability of developing a predictable and valuable practice.

XI. Arising Logical Exploration:

The expanding area of psychophysiology keeps on revealing the complexities of profound breathing and its effect on the human body. Propels in neuroimaging methods, for example, utilitarian attractive reverberation imaging (fMRI) and electroencephalography (EEG), give significant bits of knowledge into the brain associates of profound breathing practices. Research investigating the impacts of profound breathing on unambiguous medical issue, for example, nervousness problems, cardiovascular infections, and persistent agony, adds to the developing collection of proof supporting its remedial adequacy.

Conclusion:

All in all, the groundbreaking force of profound breathing activities reaches out a long ways past a basic demonstration of breathing in and breathing out. Established in old customs, approved by present day science, and embraced across societies, profound breathing arises as a flexible and open device for upgrading in general prosperity. Its effect on physiology, brain science, stress the board, mental capability, and rest quality positions profound breathing as a comprehensive way to deal with wellbeing. As people progressively perceive the significance of developing a reasonable and versatile mentality, the act of profound breathing stands as an immortal and important asset on the excursion to ideal prosperity.

Chapter6
Hand Exercise

Elated walks, an apparently straightforward yet profoundly compelling activity, have acquired prominence in different wellness and recovery settings. Whether proceeded as a feature of an exercise routine everyday practice, during non-intrusive treatment, or as a warm-up movement, situated walks offer a scope of advantages that reach out past their clear straightforwardness. In this complete investigation, we will dive into the mechanics, benefits, varieties, and uses of situated walks, revealing insight into why this apparently essential activity has turned into a staple in numerous wellness and recovery programs.

I. Grasping Situated Walks:

A. Mechanics of Situated Walks:

Situated walks include lifting and bringing down the legs on the other hand while situated on a steady surface, like a seat or seat. The development imitates the activity of walking set up, however in a situated position. The activity fundamentally connects with the muscles in the lower furthest points, zeroing in on the quadriceps, hamstrings, and lower leg muscles. Moreover, it initiates the center muscles, advancing soundness and equilibrium.

B. Legitimate Structure and Method:

Executing situated walks with appropriate structure is vital to amplify their advantages and forestall injury.

This segment will dive into the vital components of legitimate structure, including keeping an upstanding stance, adjusting the knees over the lower legs, and guaranteeing a controlled and conscious development. Accentuation will be put on the significance of drawing in the center and keeping away from exorbitant bobbing or energy.

II. Advantages of Situated Walks:

A. Reinforces Lower Body Muscles:

Situated walks give a powerful method for reinforcing the muscles in the lower body. The dull lifting and bringing down of the legs focus on the quadriceps, hamstrings, and lower leg muscles, adding to further developed leg strength and perseverance.

B. Improves Center Steadiness:

The commitment of center muscles during situated walks is instrumental in advancing center solidness. This segment will investigate how the activity enacts the abs, lower back, and oblique's, encouraging areas of strength for a steady center establishment.

C. Low-Effect Cardiovascular Activity:

Situated walks offer a low-influence cardiovascular exercise, making them reasonable for people with joint issues or those going through restoration. By lifting the pulse, this exercise adds to cardiovascular wellbeing without putting over the top weight on the joints.

D. Further develops Scope of Movement:

Standard act of situated walks can add to further developed scope of movement in the hip and knee joints. This segment will talk about how the controlled leg developments assist with keeping up with joint adaptability and forestall solidness.

III. Varieties of Situated Walks:

A. Obstruction Band Situated Walks:

Coordinating opposition groups into situated walks adds an additional aspect to the activity by giving obstruction all through the development. This variety heightens the exercise, focusing on muscles all the more really and upgrading generally strength.

B. Situated Walks with Lower leg Loads:

Lower leg loads can be consolidated to expand the opposition on the lower limits, testing the muscles further and advancing more noteworthy strength gains. This part will investigate the legitimate use of lower leg loads and their possible advantages.

C. Dependability Ball Situated Walks:

Performing situated walks on a security ball presents a component of unsteadiness, requiring more prominent commitment of the center muscles for balance. This variety focuses on the lower body as well as upgrades generally speaking strength and coordination.

IV. Utilizations of Situated Walks:

A. Wellness and Exercise Projects:

Situated walks are flexible and can be handily integrated into different wellness and exercise programs. This segment will examine how mentors and wellness devotees utilize situated walks as a feature of warm-up schedules, high-intensity exercise, or as an independent activity for lower body molding.

B. Restoration and Active recuperation:

Actual advisors frequently endorse situated walks as a component of recovery programs for people recuperating from wounds or medical procedures. The controlled and low-influence nature of the activity makes it appropriate for developing fortitude and adaptability during the recuperation cycle.

C. Work area Activities and Work environment Health:

Given the stationary idea of many positions, integrating situated walks into an everyday schedule can be helpful for office laborers. This part will investigate how work area works out, including situated walks, can add to work environment wellbeing by advancing development and decreasing the adverse consequences of drawn out sitting.

Situated walks, frequently neglected for their straightforwardness, arise as a strong activity with a large number of advantages. From reinforcing lower body muscles to improving center strength and giving a low-influence cardiovascular exercise, this exercise demonstrates its flexibility in different settings. With the incorporation of varieties and applications, situated walks become an important device for wellness lovers, recovery experts, and people looking to work on their general wellbeing and prosperity. As we keep on uncovering the profundity of its benefits, situated walks reaffirm their place as a key and open activity for people of all wellness levels

Chapter8
Sated twist

Situated turns, a crucial part of yoga and different work-out schedules, definitely stand out for their potential medical advantages. This perplexing development includes turning the chest area while situated, advancing adaptability, strength, and in general prosperity. In this extensive investigation, we dig into the beginnings of situated turns, the mechanics behind the development, and the bunch of wellbeing benefits they off.

Starting points and Advancement:

Situated turns find their foundations in antiquated rehearses like yoga and customary Indian activity frameworks. Throughout the long term, these developments have risen above social limits and become a necessary piece of different wellness regimens. The development of situated turns mirrors a combination of social impacts, mixing conventional insight with present day practice science.

Mechanics of Situated Turns:

To comprehend the advantages of situated turns, getting a handle on the mechanics of the movement is vital. Situated curves principally connect with the muscles of the center, including the oblique's, rectus abdominals, and cross over abdominals. The winding movement likewise actuates the muscles along the spine, upgrading spinal portability. Moreover, the shoulders, hips, and pelvic locale assume essential making a full-body commitment that adds to in general actual health.

Adaptability and Scope of Movement:

One of the champion benefits of situated turns lies in their capacity to improve adaptability and scope of movement. The rotational part of the development focuses on the spine, advancing gracefulness in the vertebrae. Further developed spinal adaptability supports forestalling wounds as well as works with better stance and decreases solidness related with stationary ways of life.

Center Strength and Soundness:

Situated turns are prestigious for their viability in developing center fortitude and security. The bending movement draws in the muscular strength, advancing areas of strength for a versatile center. A vigorous center, thus, adds to more readily adjust, further developed pose, and diminished hazard of back torment. The isometric compression associated with keeping up with the turn further heightens the exercise, cultivating expanded muscle perseverance.

Detoxification and Further developed Absorption:

The contorting activity in situated turns animates the organs inside the stomach hole, including the stomach related organs. This feeling can upgrade absorption by empowering the progression of stomach related squeezes and advancing peristalsis. Also, the pressure and arrival of organs during the bend might uphold the detoxification cycle, supporting the disposal of waste and poisons from the body.

Mind-Body Association:

Past the actual advantages, situated turns assume a critical part in encouraging areas of strength for a body association. The thoughtful part of yoga and comparative practices underscores care during developments. Situated turns require fixation on breath and body arrangement, advancing mental concentration and stress decrease. This psyche body collaboration adds to a general feeling of prosperity and unwinding.

Injury Anticipation and Recovery:

Situated turns are flexible and can be adjusted to various wellness levels, making them reasonable for people of different ages and states of being. The controlled idea of the development makes it a significant instrument for injury counteraction and recovery. Integrating situated turns into a balanced wellness routine can assist with tending to irregular characteristics, decrease the gamble of wounds, and help in the recuperation cycle for those with specific outer muscle issues.

Social and Otherworldly Importance:

Past their actual advantages, situated turns hold social and profound importance in different customs. In yoga, turns are frequently connected with detoxification on both a physical and enthusiastic level. The arrival of pressure and stale energy is accepted to advance an agreeable progression of prune, or life force, all through the body. Understanding the social and profound aspects adds profundity to the act of situated turns.

Conclusion:

Situated turns, with their underlying foundations in old practices and their versatility to current wellness schedules, offer an all encompassing way to deal with actual prosperity. From improving adaptability and center solidarity to encouraging areas of strength for a body association, the advantages of situated turns stretch out past the actual domain. As people keep on investigating different roads for keeping up with wellbeing and wellness, the tried and true act of situated turns remains as a demonstration of the getting through significance of old insight in the contemporary world. Embracing the specialty of bending while situated opens a passage to further developed wellbeing, essentialness, and a more profound association between the body, psyche, and soul.

Chapter9
Pelvic Tilts

Pelvic Slants: A Far reaching Manual for Figuring out, Performing, and Profiting from this Principal Exercise

Pelvic slants are a principal practice that assumes a significant part in further developing center steadiness, upgrading adaptability, and forestalling different outer muscle issues. This far reaching guide means to dig profound into the idea of pelvic slants, investigating their physical importance, various sorts, appropriate execution methods, and the horde of advantages related with their customary practice.

I. Life systems of the Pelvis:

Understanding pelvic slants starts with a grip of the pelvic life structures. The pelvis is a hard design that interfaces the spine to the lower appendages. It comprises of the sacrum, coccyx, and two hip bones, shaping a ring-like design. The pelvic slant principally includes developments of the pelvis comparable to the spine, and a reasonable comprehension of the pelvic construction is fundamental for dominating this activity.

II. Kinds of Pelvic Slants:

Front Pelvic Slant:

Definition and Causes
Impacts on Stance and Muscles
Adjustment Methods

Back Pelvic Slant:

Definition and Causes
Impacts on Stance and Muscles
Adjustment Methods
Horizontal Pelvic Slant:

Definition and Causes
Impacts on Stance and Muscles
Adjustment Strategies
Impartial Pelvic Slant:

Optimal Pelvic Arrangement
Significance for Utilitarian Development
Keeping a Nonpartisan Pelvic Slant in Day to day
Exercises

III. Advantages of Pelvic Slants:

Center Reinforcing:

Commitment of Abs
Commitment to a More grounded Center
Further developed Stance:

Tending to Postural Misalignments
Anticipation of Back Torment
Upgraded Adaptability:

Extending and Assembling Muscles around the Pelvis
Positive Effect on Generally speaking Scope of
Movement
Decreased Chance of Injury:

Settling the Lumbar Spine
Limiting Stress on Supporting Designs

Pelvic Floor Wellbeing:

Fortifying Pelvic Floor Muscles
Suggestions for People

IV. Instructions to Perform Pelvic Slants:

Prostrate Pelvic Slants:

Bit by bit Guidelines
Normal Slip-ups and How to Keep away from Them
Standing Pelvic Slants:

Legitimate Arrangement and Body Situating
Coordinating Pelvic Slants into Everyday Exercises
Situated Pelvic Slants:

Variations for Work area Laborers
Keeping up with Pelvic Wellbeing in a Stationary Way of life

V. Integrating Pelvic Slants into Work-out Schedules:

Yoga and Pilates:

Pelvic Slant Varieties in Yoga Postures
Pilates Activities for Pelvic Steadiness
Strength Preparing:

Combination into Full-Body Exercises
Focusing on Unambiguous Muscle Gatherings
Recovery and Non-intrusive treatment:

Pelvic Slants in Injury Recuperation

Tweaking Activities for Individual Necessities
VI. Normal Difficulties and Arrangements:

Conquering Snugness and Restricted Scope of Movement:

Extending and Versatility Activities
Managing Distress or Agony:

Perceiving Indications of Mistaken Structure
Looking for Proficient Direction
Keeping up with Consistency:

Ways to integrate Pelvic Slants into Everyday Daily schedule
Putting forth Sensible Objectives
VII. Conclusion:

In outline, pelvic slants offer a comprehensive way to deal with further developing center strength, upgrading adaptability, and forestalling different outer muscle issues. Whether you're a competitor, a wellness fan, or somebody hoping to resolve postural issues, incorporating pelvic slants into your routine can significantly affect your general prosperity. By grasping the life systems, dominating different slant varieties, and integrating them into assorted work-out schedules, people can open the various advantages related with this basic yet strong development.

Chapter10
Seated Side Leg Lifts

elated side leg lifts are a flexible and powerful activity that objectives different muscle gatherings, essentially zeroing in on the external thighs, hips, and oblique's. Whether you are a wellness fan hoping to reinforce your lower body or somebody looking for a low-influence practice choice, situated side leg lifts can be a significant expansion to your gym routine daily schedule. In this thorough aide, we will investigate the advantages, appropriate method, varieties, and tips to boost the viability of situated side leg lifts.

I. Advantages of Situated Side Leg Lifts:

Designated Muscle Commitment:
Situated side leg lifts principally connect with the muscles in the external thighs (abductors), hips, and oblique's. This designated actuation helps tone and reinforce these muscle gatherings, adding to further developed by and large lower body strength and steadiness.

Low-Effect Choice:
Dissimilar to some high-influence works out, situated side leg lifts are a low-influence choice, making them reasonable for people with joint issues or the individuals who favor practices that are gentler on the body. This trademark likewise goes with them a superb decision for restoration and recuperation.

Worked on Hip Adaptability:
Performing situated side leg lifts consistently can improve hip adaptability by advancing a more prominent scope of movement. This is especially valuable for people who go through extended periods sitting or have inactive ways of life.

Center Actuation:

As you lift your legs aside, your center muscles, particularly the oblique's, connect with to balance out your middle. This fortifies the center as well as improves generally equilibrium and stance.

Available Anyplace:

Situated side leg lifts should be possible anyplace, making them a helpful activity for people with occupied timetables or restricted admittance to an exercise center. All you want is a durable seat or seat.

II. Appropriate Procedure:

Set Up:

Start by sitting on a steady seat or seat with your feet level on the ground and your back straight. Put your hands on the sides of the seat for help.

Positioning:

Keep your knees twisted at a 90-degree point and your feet hip-width separated. Connect with your center muscles to keep a steady and upstanding stance.

Execution:

Lift one leg aside, keeping it straight and lined up with the ground. Hold briefly, then, at that point, lower it back down without allowing it to contact the floor. Rehash on the opposite side.

Breathing:
Breathe in as you lift your leg, and breathe out as you lower it. Center around controlled developments to augment muscle commitment.

Redundancy and Sets:
Begin with a sensible number of redundancies, like 10-15 on each side, and bit by bit increment as your solidarity gets to the next level. Hold back nothing sets.

III. Varieties of Situated Side Leg Lifts:

Opposition Groups:
Coordinate obstruction groups around your thighs to add additional opposition and heighten the exercise.

Lower leg Loads:
Tie on lower leg loads for an extra test, focusing on the muscles all the more with the utmost intensity.

Situated Side Leg Circles:
Rather than lifting the leg directly aside, perform round movements, connecting with various muscle filaments. Fix your legs completely, lifting them aside, to connect with the muscles another way and increment trouble.

IV. Tips for Greatest Adequacy:

Mind-Body Association:
Center around the muscles you are focusing on and keep major areas of strength for a body association all through the activity.

Slow Movement:
Begin with an agreeable scope of movement and progressively increment it as your adaptability and strength get to the next level.

Consistency is Critical:
For ideal outcomes, integrate situated side leg lifts into your normal work-out daily practice and remain steady after some time.

Pay attention to Your Body:
Focus on any distress or agony, and adjust the activity depending on the situation. Talk with a wellness expert or medical services supplier on the off chance that you have any worries.

Join with Different Activities:
Incorporate situated side leg lifts as a component of a complete lower body exercise to guarantee adjusted muscle improvement.

Conclusion:

Situated side leg lifts offer a huge number of advantages, from designated muscle commitment to further developed adaptability and center strength. By dominating the appropriate strategy, investigating varieties, and integrating steady practice into your wellness schedule, you can open the maximum capacity of this adaptable activity. Whether you are a wellness beginner or an accomplished fan, situated side leg lifts give an important device to improving your lower body strength, soundness, and in general prosperity

Chapter 11
Chest Stretches

Chest extends assume an essential part in keeping up with in general adaptability and portability. Whether you're a competitor, wellness lover, or somebody looking for help from an inactive way of life, integrating chest extends into your routine can achieve various advantages. This extensive aide will dig into the significance of chest extends, the life systems of the chest, and give an itemized rundown of compelling chest stretches to improve your scope of movement and lessen muscle pressure.

Understanding the Significance of Chest Stretches:

Postural Improvement:

Chest stretches can assist with balancing the impacts of unfortunate stance, which is a typical issue in the present stationary way of life. Extending the chest muscles opens up the front of the body, advancing an upstanding stance and diminishing the gamble of creating adjusted shoulders and a slouched back.

Improved Scope of Movement:

Integrating chest extends into your routine can work on the adaptability and portability of the shoulder joints. This expanded scope of movement is especially valuable for competitors engaged with sports that require above developments, like swimming, tennis, and weightlifting.

Reducing Muscle Pressure:

The chest muscles, especially the pectorals major and minor, can turn out to be tight and add to chest area inconvenience. Ordinary chest extending can mitigate muscle pressure, lessening firmness and advancing unwinding in the chest and shoulder area.

Injury Anticipation:

Adaptable and flexible muscles are less inclined to wounds. By consistently integrating chest extends into your wellness schedule, you can forestall muscle awkward nature, lessen the gamble of strains, and upgrade in general solid flexibility.

Life structures of the Chest Muscles:

Understanding the life structures of the chest muscles is fundamental for successful extending. The essential muscles focused on during chest extends include:

Pectorals Major:

The biggest muscle in the chest, the pectorals major, comprises of two sections: the clavicle head (upper chest) and the sternal head (lower chest). Extending the two bits is indispensable for thorough chest adaptability.

Pectorals Minor:

Situated underneath the pectorals major, the pectorals minor adds to bear development. Extending this muscle is pivotal for delivering strain in the shoulder district.
Successful Chest Stretches:

Entryway Chest Stretch:

Stand in an entryway with your arms bowed at a 90-degree point. Put your lower arms on the door jamb and incline forward, feeling the stretch across your chest.

Chest Opener Stretch:

Sit or stand tall, interweave your fingers despite your good faith, and fix your arms. Lift your arms somewhat, opening your chest and pressing your shoulder bones together.

Wall Chest Stretch:

Face a wall and broaden one arm at shoulder level, putting your palm on the wall with fingers pointing in reverse. Gradually dismiss your body from the wall to feel a profound stretch in the chest.

Cross-Body Arm Stretch:

Bring your right arm across your chest and utilize your passed available to pull it closer delicately. Hold the stretch and afterward switch sides.

Kid's Posture with Chest Opener:

Begin in a bowing position, sit out of sorts, and expand your arms forward. Walk your hands aside, feeling the stretch at the edge of your middle and chest.

Conclusion:

Integrating chest extends into your standard wellness routine is significant for keeping up with ideal adaptability, further developing stance, and forestalling wounds. By understanding the significance of chest extends and focusing on the key muscles included, you can upgrade your general prosperity and partake in a more useful and torment free chest area. Make these stretches a steady piece of your everyday practice to encounter the drawn out advantages of expanded chest adaptability and portability.

Chapter 12
Seated rowing

Situated paddling is an exceptionally viable and flexible activity that frames a necessary piece of solidarity preparing schedules. Whether you're a carefully prepared rec center participant or a novice, integrating situated lines into your gym routine can yield various advantages for generally wellness and muscle improvement. In this complete aide, we will dive into the complexities of situated paddling, covering its procedure, benefits, and different varieties to assist you with upgrading your preparation.

I. Grasping Situated Paddling Procedure:

Arrangement and Hardware:
Situated paddling commonly requires a link machine or a paddling machine. Begin by changing the seat level and guaranteeing that your feet are safely put on the hassocks. Handle the handle with an overhand grasp, keeping your hands marginally more extensive than shoulder-width separated.

Body Position:
Keep an upstanding stance all through the activity. Connect with your center, hold your shoulders back, and try not to adjust your back. This legitimate body arrangement guarantees that you focus on the expected muscles and decrease the gamble of injury.

Pulling Movement:

Start the development by withdrawing your shoulder bones and pulling the handle towards your lower chest. Center around pressing your back muscles as you arrive at the completely contracted position. Control the drop as you return the handle to the beginning position, keeping up with opposition all through the whole scope of movement.

Breathing Strategy:

Coordinate your breathing with the development. Breathe in as you broaden your arms and breathe out during the pulling stage. This balances out your center and upgrades by and large control during the activity.

II. Advantages of Situated Paddling:

Muscle Commitment:

Situated paddling essentially focuses on the muscles of the upper back, including the latissimus dorsa, rhomboids, and traps. Moreover, it draws in the biceps and lower arms, giving a complete chest area exercise.

Further developed Stance:

Ordinary fuse of situated columns into your routine adds to all the more likely stance. Reinforcing the muscles answerable for scapular withdrawal advances a more upstanding position and lessens the probability of creating adjusted shoulders.

Joint Wellbeing:

Situated paddling is a compound activity that includes different joints. This assists improve with jointing steadiness and adaptability, cultivating generally joint wellbeing and diminishing the gamble of wounds related with irregular characteristics or shortcomings.

Adaptability for All Wellness Levels:

Situated paddling can be handily altered to oblige different wellness levels. Changing the obstruction, utilizing different hold varieties, or integrating one-sided developments permits fledglings and high level lifters the same to fit the activity to their particular requirements.

III. Situated Paddling Varieties:

Wide Hold Situated Column:

Extending your grasp on the handle puts more accentuation on the external last, assisting with accomplishing a more extensive back. This variety likewise draws in the back deltoids and trees major.

Close Grasp Situated Column:

Uniting your hands focuses on the center of the back, explicitly the rhomboids. This variety can add to a more characterized and etched back appearance.

Single-Arm Situated Line:

Playing out the situated column with each arm in turn upgrades one-sided strength and addresses muscle awkward nature. It additionally requests more prominent center security as your body attempts to oppose turn.

Turn around Hold Situated Line:

Changing your hold to an underhand position moves the concentration to the lower last and biceps. This variety gives an interesting test and can be useful for those hoping to change up their daily practice.

Conclusion:

Situated paddling remains as a central activity with a huge number of advantages for people chasing after strength, muscle improvement, and by and large wellness. Dominating the appropriate strategy, figuring out the related advantages, and investigating different situated paddling varieties can essentially improve your preparation experience. Whether you're expecting to work on your stance, shape your back, or reinforce your chest area, situated paddling merits a noticeable spot in your exercise routine everyday practice.

Chapter 13
Seated knee

Ext Situated knee expansions, a famous practice in the domain of solidarity preparing and recovery, include expanding the knee joint against opposition while situated. This exercise basically focuses on the quadriceps muscles, giving different advantages to people meaning to upgrade lower appendage strength, work on joint steadiness, or recuperate from knee wounds. Notwithstanding, similar to any activity, situated knee augmentations accompany their own arrangement of contemplations, including likely dangers and contraindications. This article dives into the complexities of situated knee expansions, investigating their advantages, legitimate execution, varieties, and possible dangers to give an exhaustive comprehension of this activity.

Advantages of Situated Knee Augmentations:

Separation of Quadriceps Muscles:
Situated knee expansions principally focus on the quadriceps muscles, which comprise of four particular muscles situated on the facade of the thigh. This segregation considers an engaged and serious exercise, supporting muscle improvement and definition.

Joint Steadiness and Usefulness:
The activity draws in the knee joint, advancing security and utilitarian strength. Reinforcing the quadriceps is pivotal for exercises like strolling, running, and climbing

steps, adding to generally joint wellbeing and versatility.

Recovery Purposes:

Situated knee augmentations are frequently integrated into recovery programs for people recuperating from knee wounds or medical procedures. The controlled idea of the activity takes into account progressive reinforcing of the quadriceps without putting unreasonable weight on the recuperating joint.

Adjustable Obstruction:

Situated knee augmentations can be performed with different opposition levels, including body weight, obstruction groups, or machine loads. This versatility makes the activity reasonable for people at various wellness levels and those with shifting levels of solidarity.

Legitimate Execution of Situated Knee Augmentations:

Right Seating Position:

Start by changing the seat level to guarantee legitimate arrangement of the knee joint with the machine's turn point. The backrest ought to offer help without causing hyperextension of the lower back.

Foot Situation:

Position your feet on the footstool, guaranteeing they are hip-width separated. The toes ought to point forward or somewhat outward, and the knees ought to be in accordance with the machine's turn point.

Scope of Movement:

Execute the development by expanding your knees until your legs are straight without locking the joints. Control the drop to the beginning situation to amplify muscle commitment and limit weight on the knee joints.

Varieties of Situated Knee Augmentations:

One-sided Situated Knee Augmentations:

Play out the activity each leg in turn to address muscle lopsided characteristics and advance one-sided strength improvement.

Two-sided Situated Knee Augmentations with Groups: Consolidate opposition groups to add variable obstruction all through the scope of movement, heightening the exercise and testing balancing out muscles.

Isometric Holds:

Present isometric holds at the highest point of the development to improve muscle perseverance and advance more noteworthy time under pressure.

Possible Dangers and Contemplations:

Patellofemoral Stress:

Extreme stacking during situated knee expansions can put weight on the Patellofemoral joint, possibly adding to knee agony or uneasiness, particularly in people with prior knee conditions.

Back Strain:

Unfortunate seating stance or hyperextension of the lower back can prompt back strain. It is essential to keep an impartial spine position all through the activity.

Hazard of Hyperextension:

Locking the knees at the highest point of the development might prompt hyperextension, expanding the gamble of injury. Center around controlled, smooth motions without completely locking the knee joints.

Contraindications:

People with specific knee conditions, like patellar tendinitis or tendon wounds, ought to counsel a medical care proficient prior to integrating situated knee expansions into their gym routine daily practice.

Conclusion:

Situated knee expansions offer a plenty of advantages, from quadriceps muscle improvement to joint security and restoration purposes. When executed with legitimate structure and thought of individual restrictions, this exercise can be an important expansion to a balanced work out schedule. In any case, understanding the likely dangers and contraindications is fundamental to guarantee a protected and viable exercise. Likewise with any activity, people ought to talk with wellness experts or medical care suppliers to decide the reasonableness of situated knee augmentations in light of their particular requirements and wellbeing status.

Chapter 14
Toe taps

the huge domain of dance, where development is a language and articulation takes heap frames, the humble yet enrapturing toe tap stands apart as a cadenced accentuation mark. From its foundations in customary moves to its cutting edge variations across different sorts, toe taps have persevered through everyday hardship as well as developed into a powerful articulation of creativity and development.

Verifiable Roots:

Toe taps find their beginnings in customary dance shapes that range across societies and mainland's. In the rich embroidery of dance history, these apparently basic foot developments play had a critical impact in both people and old style moves. From the percussive footwork in Irish step moving to the mind boggling designs in Spanish flamenco, toe taps have been a crucial component, adding both hear-able and visual aspects to the exhibitions.

Development in Tap Dance:

The most unmistakable development of toe taps can be seen in the domain of tap dance, a type that has taken the musical capability of footwork higher than ever. Rising up out of the combination of African, Irish, and English dance customs in North America, tap dance turned into a social peculiarity in the mid twentieth hundred years. The toe tap, alongside the heel tap, turned into the heartbeat of this musical dance structure.

Tap artists, from legends like Bill Robinson to contemporary craftsmen like Savior Glover, have raised toe takes advantage of a work of art that goes past simple percussion. The accuracy and enunciation of the toe tap have become key to the expressive language of tap artists, permitting them to make mind boggling rhythms and songs with their feet. The development of tap dance grandstands how toe taps have changed from utilitarian footwork to a refined and creative language of their own.

Social Varieties:

Past the domains of tap dance, toe taps keep on assuming a huge part in different social dance structures. In Indian traditional dance, for instance, the "rite" or unadulterated dance part frequently consolidates unpredictable footwork, including toe taps, to make cadenced examples that supplement the music. Essentially, in African dance customs, toe taps are used as a feature of the complex polyrhythmic structures that characterize the developments.

Present day Understandings:

In the contemporary dance scene, choreographers and artists have embraced toe taps for of adding surface and intricacy to their works. The flexibility of toe taps permits artists to try different things with various styles, mixing customary procedures with present day developments. This combination of old and new makes a unique transaction among custom and development, giving toe taps a new and pertinent presence in the steadily advancing universe of dance.

Advancement Past Dance:

The impact of toe taps reaches out past the limits of dance, transforming other fine arts also. Performers have integrated toe takes advantage of their syntheses, involving them as percussive components to add an exceptional layer of sound to their music. The combination of tap dance and unrecorded music, where toe taps synchronize with instruments, represents the consistent incorporation of this cadenced strategy into different creative articulations.

Instructive Importance:

Toe taps likewise hold instructive worth, filling in as a major structure block for yearning artists. Dominating the complexities of toe taps requires discipline, coordination, and a comprehension of beat. Dance teachers frequently use toe tap activities to show understudies the significance of accuracy in development and the subtleties of musicality, cultivating a profound appreciation for the association among dance and music.

Conclusion:

Toe taps, when established in the conventional moves of different societies, have developed into a flexible and powerful component in the realm of dance and then some. From their verifiable importance in tap dance to their presence in contemporary movement, toe taps keep on enthralling crowds and specialists the same. As we praise the cadenced language of toe taps, we witness an immortal dance among custom and development, where the straightforward demonstration of tapping one's toes turns into a significant articulation of human innovativeness.

Toe taps, an apparently straightforward and honest activity, have found their direction into different wellness schedules, dance practices, and recovery programs. Regardless of their direct appearance, toe taps envelop a large number of advantages, from upgrading cardiovascular wellness to further developing coordination and equilibrium. This complete investigation dives into the workmanship and science behind toe taps, revealing insight into their diverse nature and the effect they can have on our general prosperity.

Verifiable Roots:

The starting points of toe taps can be followed back to customary dance structures where complex footwork and musical developments assumed a vital part. These early practices established the groundwork for the reconciliation of toe takes advantage of current wellness and recovery programs. Over the long haul, toe taps have developed from a social articulation to a flexible activity with various applications.

Fundamental Strategy:

Toe taps include a basic yet viable development design. To play out a fundamental toe tap, a singular takes one foot off the ground and delicately taps the toes on an assigned surface, shifting back and forth between feet. This monotonous activity draws in different muscle gatherings, including the lower appendages and center, making it an effective full-body work out.

Cardiovascular Advantages:

One of the essential benefits of toe taps lies in their capacity to hoist the pulse, adding to worked on cardiovascular wellness. The cadenced idea of the activity reenacts the impacts of vigorous exercises, making it an available choice for those looking to upgrade their perseverance and endurance.

Coordination and Equilibrium:

Toe taps request a serious level of coordination between the upper and lower body. As people lift and tap their toes, they connect with the center muscles and challenge their equilibrium. Ordinary act of toe taps can prompt better coordination and upgraded proprioception, which is urgent for forestalling falls and wounds.

Versatility in Work out schedules:

One of the astounding highlights of toe taps is their versatility to different wellness levels and settings. Whether integrated into intense cardio exercise (HIIT), dance schedules, or recovery works out, toe taps can be altered to suit various necessities. This flexibility has added to their prominence among wellness aficionados, competitors, and medical care experts the same.

Recovery Applications:

Toe taps assume a critical part in recovery programs for people recuperating from wounds, especially those influencing the lower furthest points. The controlled and low-influence nature of the activity takes into consideration designated muscle actuation without overburdening harmed regions. Actual advisors frequently incorporate toe taps to further develop strength, adaptability, and scope of movement during the recuperation interaction.

Mental Advantages:

Past the actual angles, toe taps additionally offer mental advantages. The need to synchronize developments and keep a reliable beat cultivates mental concentration and focus. Integrating toe takes advantage of a wellness routine can act as a careful activity, advancing the association among psyche and body.

Varieties and Movements:

To forestall dreariness and consistently challenge the body, different toe tap varieties and movements can be presented. These may incorporate integrating extra arm developments, speeding up taps, or playing out the activity on a temperamental surface. These varieties not just add a component of energy to the exercise yet in addition target different muscle bunches for a more thorough preparation experience.

Joining into Dance:

Given their verifiable roots in dance, toe taps consistently coordinate into dance schedules across various kinds. From tap moving to current dance, the joining of toe taps improves footwork accuracy and adds dynamic components to movement. Artists frequently use toe taps as a basic structure block for additional mind boggling developments and groupings.

Conclusion:

All in all, toe taps epitomize the combination of custom and advancement in the domain of wellness and dance. From their unassuming starting points in social practices to their boundless use in restoration and contemporary exercises, toe taps have demonstrated to be a flexible and successful activity. As we keep on investigating the perplexing connection among development and prosperity, the effortlessness of toe taps remains as a demonstration of the significant effect that an apparently essential activity can have on our physical and psychological well-being.

Chapter 15
Seated hamstring stretch

Extending is an essential part of any exhaustive wellness standard, adding to further developed adaptability, scope of movement, and in general outer muscle wellbeing. Among the horde of extending works out, the situated hamstring stretch stands apart as a powerful method for focusing on and upgrade the adaptability of the hamstrings. This complete investigation digs into the life structures of the hamstrings, the advantages of the situated hamstring stretch, and different procedures to ideally play out this stretch.

I. Life systems of the Hamstrings:

The hamstrings are a gathering of three muscles situated at the rear of the thigh: the biceps femora's, semitendinosus, and semimembranosus. These muscles assume a vital part in hip expansion and knee flexion, making them fundamental for exercises like strolling, running, and bouncing. Understanding the life structures of the hamstrings is essential to valuing the meaning of extending and keeping up with their adaptability.

Biceps Femora's: This muscle is partitioned into two heads - the long head and the short head. Both add to knee flexion and hip expansion.

Semitendinosus: Situated medially, this muscle supports knee flexion and hip expansion.

Semimembranosus: Arranged further than the other two, this muscle additionally adds to knee flexion and hip augmentation.

II. Advantages of Situated Hamstring Stretch:

The situated hamstring stretch offers a horde of advantages, impacting the hamstrings as well as the by and large outer muscle framework and general prosperity.

Further developed Adaptability: Customary act of the situated hamstring stretch upgrades the adaptability of the hamstrings, considering a more prominent scope of movement in ordinary exercises.

Injury Counteraction:
Adaptable hamstrings can add to forestalling wounds, especially strains and tears, by advancing better muscle versatility and joint capability.

Decreased Lower Back Agony:
Tight hamstrings can add to bring down back torment. The situated hamstring stretch mitigates this uneasiness by delivering pressure in the hamstring muscles, accordingly lessening burden on the lower back.

Upgraded Stance: Adaptable hamstrings assume a significant part in keeping up with great stance. Integrating the situated hamstring stretch into a routine can add to a more upstanding and adjusted pose.

Further developed Dissemination: Extending invigorates blood stream to the extended muscles, advancing better course. This expanded blood stream can assist in lessening with muscling irritation and speeding up the recuperation cycle.

III. Methods for Situated Hamstring Stretch:

Playing out the situated hamstring stretch accurately is critical to augment its advantages and limit the gamble of injury. Here, we investigate different methods to really execute this stretch.

Situated Ahead Twist:

Sit on the floor with your legs broadened straight before you.
Pivot at your hips and incline forward, going after your toes.
Keep your back straight and try not to adjust your spine.
Hold the stretch for 15-30 seconds, breathing profoundly.

Situated Single-Leg Hamstring Stretch:

Sit with one leg broadened straight and the underside of the other foot against the inward thigh of the drawn out leg.
Pivot at the hips and reach toward the toes of the drawn out leg.
Keep a straight back and feel the stretch along the rear of the lengthy leg.
Hold for 15-30 seconds and switch legs.

Situated Wide-Leg Forward Twist:

Sit with your legs spread wide separated.
Pivot at the hips and incline forward, going after the floor.
Keep your back straight and feel the stretch in the internal thighs and hamstrings.
Hold for 15-30 seconds, breathing profoundly.

Situated Hamstring Stretch with a Band:

Sit with your legs broadened and circle an opposition band around the wads of your feet.
Hold the finishes of the band with your hands.
Pivot at the hips and incline forward, utilizing the band to extend the stretch.
Hold for 15-30 seconds, keeping a straight back.

The situated hamstring stretch arises as an adaptable and successful activity for improving hamstring adaptability and advancing in general outer muscle wellbeing. Figuring out the life systems of the hamstrings, perceiving the horde advantages of this stretch, and dominating different strategies for its execution furnishes people with the information to actually integrate this stretch into their wellness schedules. Ordinary act of the situated hamstring stretch not just adds to further developed adaptability and injury counteraction yet in addition cultivates a feeling of prosperity by advancing better stance and diminishing muscle strain. Similarly as with any activity, it is prudent to talk with a medical services proficient or wellness master prior to integrating new stretches into a daily schedule, particularly for people with previous ailments or wounds.

The situated hamstring stretch is an essential activity that objectives the muscles at the rear of the thigh, advancing adaptability, lessening muscle pressure, and improving generally lower body portability. Whether you're a competitor, wellness aficionado, or somebody hoping to work on their adaptability, understanding the advantages and appropriate procedures of the situated hamstring stretch can contribute essentially to your general prosperity.

I. Life structures of the Hamstrings:

Prior to diving into the situated hamstring stretch, understanding the life structures of the hamstrings is urgent. The hamstrings comprise of three essential muscles - the biceps femora's, semitendinosus, and semimembranosus. These muscles assume a crucial part in different lower body developments, including strolling, running, and bouncing. Extending the hamstrings is fundamental for keeping up with their adaptability and forestalling wounds.

II. Advantages of the Situated Hamstring Stretch:

Further developed Adaptability:

The situated hamstring stretch is eminent for improving adaptability in the hamstrings, which can decidedly affect your general scope of movement.

Expanded adaptability can prompt superior execution in different proactive tasks, like games and weightlifting.

Decreased Muscle Pressure:

Stationary ways of life, delayed sitting, and extraordinary proactive tasks can add to muscle pressure in the hamstrings.
The situated hamstring stretch mitigates muscle strain, advancing unwinding and diminishing the gamble of wounds.

Counteraction of Lower Back Agony:

Tight hamstrings are frequently connected to bring down back torment. Consistently integrating the situated hamstring stretch into your routine can add to lightening or forestalling lower back distress.

Upgraded Stance:

Adaptable hamstrings assume a critical part in keeping up with legitimate stance. Extending these muscles consistently can help in accomplishing and keeping up with great postural arrangement.

Injury Avoidance:

Adaptable hamstrings are less inclined to wounds, like strains and tears. Counting the situated hamstring stretch in your warm-up routine can add to injury counteraction during proactive tasks.

III. Appropriate Method for the Situated Hamstring Stretch

Start by sitting on the floor with your legs reached out before you.
Sit tall, drawing in your center muscles to help your spine.

Execution:

Breathe in as you stretch your spine, arriving at your arms above.
Breathe out and pivot at your hips, inclining forward from your abdomen.
Keep your back straight as you reach toward your toes.

Foot Situating:

Flex your feet to really focus on the hamstrings more.
Guarantee your knees are straight however not locked.

Agreeable Stretch:

Just go to the extent that you can while keeping an agreeable stretch.
Abstain from skipping, which can prompt wounds.

Hold and Relax:

Hold the stretch for 15-30 seconds, breathing profoundly to unwind into the position.
Rehash the stretch 2-3 times, step by step expanding the length as your adaptability gets to the next leve

Utilizing Props:

Place a yoga tie around the bottoms of your feet to serenely assist with arriving at your toes.
Utilize a rolled-up towel under your knees for added help.
Situated Hamstring Stretch with a Bend:

Add a curve to the stretch by arriving at one arm towards the contrary foot, advancing extra adaptability in the spine.

Dynamic Situated Hamstring Stretch:

Play out a powerful variant by delicately shaking this way and that in the stretch to continuously further develop adaptability.

V. Safety measures and Contraindications:

Abstain from Overextending:

While it's fundamental for challenge your adaptability, try not to drive your body excessively far to forestall wounds.
Injury or Distress:

On the off chance that you have a hamstring injury or experience torment during the stretch, talk with a medical services proficient prior to proceeding.

Warm-up:

Play out a light warm-up prior to endeavoring the situated hamstring stretch to set up your muscles for the street.

Integrating the situated hamstring stretch into your wellness routine can achieve a large number of advantages, going from upgraded adaptability and diminished muscle pressure to further developed stance and injury counteraction. By understanding the appropriate method and taking into account changes in light of your singular requirements, you can fit this stretch to supplement your general wellness objectives. Make the situated hamstring stretch a reliable piece of your daily schedule, and witness the positive effect it can have on your lower body portability and generally speaking prosperity

Practice guide

First and foremost, attempt each exercise 2 or multiple times and gradually increment the
redundancies as you develop fortitude and certainty.
For instance, in a couple
of days you could rehash each exercise multiple times, stirring up to 10
reiterations in two or multi week's time.

Heel slides

1. Lying on your back.
2. Twist your knee to the furthest extent that you would be able
then fix.
3. Rehash multiple times.
4. Rehash with your other leg.

1. Lying in bed, attempt to fix your knee however much you can.
2. Push your knee down
delicately against the bed.
3. Hold for 5 seconds then
unwind
4. Rehash multiple times for every leg

Straight leg raises

1. Lying on your back with one leg straight and the other leg twisted.
2. Practice your straight leg by pulling the toes up, fixing the
knee and lifting the leg 4
creeps off the bed.
3. Hold approx. 5 seconds and
gradually unwind.
4. Rehash multiple times.

Bed and Situated Activities 3

Arm Swings

1. Sit tall away from the rear of the seat.
2. Put your feet level on the floor underneath your knees
3. Twist your elbows and swing your arms
from the shoulder
4. Fabricate a beat that is agreeable for you
5. Go on for 30 seconds

Seat Walking

1. Sit tall away from the rear of the seat
2. Hold the sides of the seat
3. On the other hand lift your feet and spot them down with control.
4. Work to a beat that is agreeable for you
5. Go on for 30 seconds

Neck Stretch
1. Delicately bring your right ear down to your right shoulder, hold for 5
2. Get back to the middle
3. Delicately bring your left ear down on your left side shoulder, hold for 5
4. Rehash multiple times
Bed and Situated Activities 4
Heel raises (situated)
1. Sit tall away from the rear of your seat
2. Lift your heels up off the ground. Ensure your toes stay on the ground
3. Rehash multiple times
Front knee strengtheners
Knee fortifying activities will assist you with keeping up with strength in the muscle at the front of your leg.
To reinforce the knee:
1. Sit solidly toward the rear of a seat, keep your shoulders down and keep up with great stance.
2. Regardless of a lower leg weight, gradually expand your leg before you.
3. Rehash up to multiple times on every leg.

Figuring out the Hamstrings:

Prior to diving into situated hamstring extends, it's vital to comprehend the muscles you're focusing on. The hamstrings comprise of three essential muscles situated at the rear of the thigh: the biceps femora's, semitendinosus, and semimembranosus. These muscles assume a crucial part in hip expansion and knee flexion, making them fundamental for exercises like strolling, running, and bouncing.

Methods for Situated Hamstring Stretches:

Basic Situated Stretch:

Sit on the floor with your legs expanded straight before you.
Pivot at your hips and reach forward toward your toes.
Keep your back straight and try not to adjust your spine.
Hold the stretch for 15-30 seconds, bit by bit expanding the span over the long run.
Situated Ahead Twist
Sit with your legs expanded and somewhat separated.
Breathe in as you protract your spine, and breathe out as you pivot at the hips, coming to advance.
Expect to get a handle on your feet or shins, keeping a delicate stretch.
Hold for 20-40 seconds, breathing profoundly to build unwinding and adaptability.

Butterfly Stretch:

Sit with the bottoms of your feet together, framing a precious stone shape with your legs.
Hold your feet and delicately press your knees towards the floor.
Keep an upstanding stance and hold the stretch for 20-30 seconds.

Wide-Legged Forward Twist:

Sit with your legs spread wide separated.
Pivot at your hips and reach forward, planning to contact the floor.
Save your back straight and hold the stretch for 20-40 seconds.

Advantages of Situated Hamstring Stretches:

Further developed Adaptability:

Ordinary act of situated hamstring extends expands the adaptability of the hamstrings, considering a more prominent scope of movement in day to day exercises.

Diminished Muscle Snugness:

Sitting for stretched out periods can prompt hamstring snugness. Situated extends assist with easing this snugness, diminishing the gamble of uneasiness and injury.

Upgraded Stance:

Fortifying and extending the hamstrings adds to more readily act by advancing a reasonable arrangement of the pelvis and spine.

Adaptable hamstrings are less inclined to wounds, like strains or tears. Integrating these stretches into your routine can be a preventive measure for competitors and people with a functioning way of life.
Normal Errors to Stay away from:

Adjusting the Back:

One of the most well-known botches is adjusting the back during situated extends. This can strain the lower back and lessen the adequacy of the stretch.
Compelling the Stretch:

Try not to compel your body into a stretch. All things being equal, slide into it step by step to forestall injury and permit your muscles to adjust.
Ignoring Warm-Up:

Performing situated hamstring extends without a legitimate warm-up can prompt muscle strain. Incorporate light oxygen consuming action or dynamic stretches prior to taking part in situated extends.
Overlooking Torment:

While extending could cause gentle distress, it ought to never be excruciating. Assuming you experience sharp agony, back out of the stretch quickly to forestall injury.

Situated hamstring extends are significant for anybody trying to upgrade adaptability, forestall wounds, and advance in general muscle wellbeing. By integrating these methods into your daily practice and being aware of normal mix-ups, you can open the various advantages of situated hamstring extends. Keep in mind, consistency is critical, and over the long haul, you'll encounter expanded adaptability and worked on prosperity.

The situated knee stretch principally centers around extending the muscles encompassing the knee joint, including the quadriceps, hamstrings, and lower leg muscles. This exercise is especially helpful for people trying to further develop adaptability, ease knee uneasiness, and upgrade generally lower body portability.

II. Advantages of the Situated Knee Stretch

Further developed Adaptability: Participating in ordinary situated knee stretches can altogether upgrade the adaptability of the muscles around the knee joint, prompting further developed scope of movement.
Joint Wellbeing: The situated knee stretch assists in advancing with jointing wellbeing by diminishing firmness and expanding blood stream to the knee region. This, thus, helps with forestalling wounds and keeping up with ideal joint capability.
Easing of Knee Inconvenience: People encountering gentle knee inconvenience or firmness might find help through the delicate and controlled developments of the situated knee stretch.

Upgraded Stance:
 Fortifying and extending the muscles around the knee can decidedly influence generally lower body arrangement, adding to all the more likely stance.

III. Legitimate Execution of the Situated Knee Stretch

Adhere to these bit by bit guidelines to guarantee legitimate execution of the situated knee stretch:

Track down an Agreeable Situated Position: Sit on a mat with your legs stretched out before you. Guarantee your spine is straight, and your shoulders are loose.

Twist One Knee
: Twist one knee and bring the bottom of your foot toward the inward thigh of the contrary leg.
: Guarantee that your bowed knee is pointing towards the side, making an agreeable plot for your hip and knee joints.

Delicate Forward Lean:
 Gradually and delicately incline forward from your hips, coming to toward your toes. Keep your back straight and try not to adjust your spine.

Hold the Stretch
: Hold the stretch for 15-30 seconds, feeling a delicate draw in the muscles around the knee. Inhale profoundly and unwind into the stretch.

Switch Sides
: Rehash the stretch on the other leg to keep up with equilibrium and evenness.

IV. Varieties of the Situated Knee Stretch

Situated Knee Embrace: While situated, embrace one knee towards your chest, making a stretch toward the rear of the knee and the hip. Switch legs and rehash.

Situated Knee Circle: Broaden one leg and turn your lower leg in round movements. This variety assists in advancing versatility and adaptability in the knee with jointing. Situated Butterfly Stretch: Sit with the bottoms of your feet together, permitting your knees to drop outward. Hold your feet with your hands and tenderly press your knees towards the floor.

V. Safeguards and Tips

Warm-up: Continuously play out a light warm-up prior to taking part in situated knee stretches to set up the muscles for adaptability works out.

Delicate Developments:
 Try not to compel your body into the stretch. All things considered, center around delicate and controlled developments to forestall injury.

Consultation
: People with existing knee wounds or persistent circumstances ought to talk with a medical services proficient or a wellness master prior to integrating the situated knee stretch into their everyday practice.

conclusion

The situated knee stretch is a flexible and open activity that holds various advantages for people of all wellness levels. Whether you're a carefully prepared competitor hoping to upgrade execution or somebody looking for help from knee distress, coordinating this stretch into your routine can add to further developed adaptability, joint wellbeing, and in general prosperity. Make sure to move toward the situated knee stretch with care, and partake in the excursion of opening the capability of your lower body.